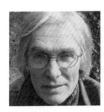

ARE TI
in 1952. *
he has ɛ
medicine,   ...e,
osteopathy   ... Since 1981
he has run ɛ ... vate holistic practice in
Sandefjord, Norway, for the healing of small animals
and horses, as well as people. He has lectured widely,
specializing in veterinary acupuncture, and has published dozens of scholarly articles. In 1984 he started to
treat cancer patients, both human and animals, and this
work has been the focus of much of his recent research.
He is the author of *Demons and Healing* (2018), *Experiences from the Threshold and Beyond* (2019) and *Spiritual
Translocation* (2020, all Temple Lodge) and several other
books on complementary medicine published in various
languages.

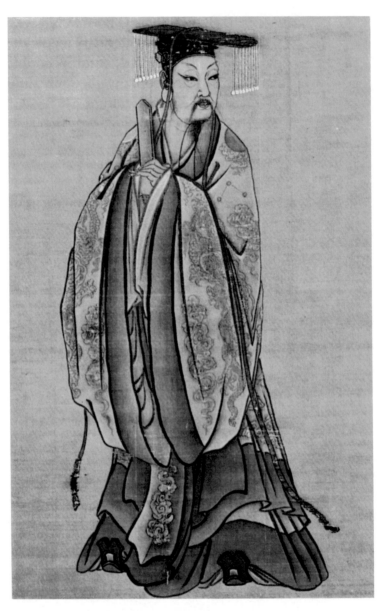

King Yu of Xia as imagined by Song Dynasty painter Ma Lin.
Hanging scroll (National Palace Museum, Taipei)

THE LUCIFER DECEPTION

The Yellow Emperor Unveiled

Secrets of Traditional Oriental Medicine

Are Simeon Thoresen, DVM

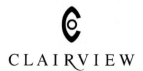

CLAIRVIEW

Dedicated to All Who Seek to Heal and Understand

Clairview Books Ltd.
Russet, Sandy Lane,
West Hoathly,
W. Sussex RH19 4QQ

www.clairviewbooks.com

Published by Clairview Books 2020

A CIP catalogue record for this book is available from the British Library

ISBN 978 1 912992 17 1

Cover by Morgan Creative featuring image of the Yellow Emperor, mural painting from Han dynasty
Typeset by Symbiosys Technologies, Vishakapatnam, India
Printed and bound by 4Edge Ltd, Essex

Contents

Author's Note

A brief summary of my background will enable the reader to better understand this book. Very early in my life I developed a kind of clairvoyance, so that now and then I could observe spiritual beings, especially those belonging to the elements of water and wind.

I then educated myself in various healing modalities, such as agronomy, veterinary science, homeopathy, herbalism, traditional Chinese medicine, acupuncture, anthroposophic medicine, etc. – the list is long.

Very early in my work I observed that pets always adapted to the pathological structure of their owners, and after three weeks they became almost the same. I also observed that the etheric bodies* of people who lived together became similar after three years, especially if they slept in the same room. They also formed

---

* Rudolf Steiner described and taught that the human body is made up of four sheaths. The first is the physical body made up of substances gathered from (and that return to) the organic world. The second level is the life force, also called the etheric body, which is held in common with all living creatures, including plants. It provides the living formative forces that sculpt the individual physical body. This etheric body is closely connected to its physical counterpart and stays with it during sleep. The third level is termed the astral body and relates to consciousness, in common with all animals. It consists of soul forces that fine-tune the physical. The astral body contains the senses and is the instrument of emotions and feelings. Finally, the fourth layer, called the 'I', is the ego which anchors the faculty of self-awareness and free will unique to human beings. It is associated with the spirit, that is higher than the soul, and conveys divine human selfhood that gives us the capacity for transformation. The 'I' is immortal and reincarnates.

identical pathological structures, as I found by means of pulse diagnosis.*

The way I use pulse diagnosis enables me to gain entry to the spiritual world, and there I can diagnose all the energetic and spiritual changes in humans and animals.

In my effort to understand diseases I soon observed that the pathological information, as well as the etheric information, lives as elemental beings within our bodies, and that these elemental, pathological beings – which I prefer to call demons – can 'jump' over from one person to another, or to an animal.

In treating diseases, when using herbs, homeopathy or acupuncture, these demons are actively transferred within three days to other beings – or within three weeks using allopathic medicine. I spent twenty years trying to find healing techniques that could stop this transloca-tion, and finally found a method that worked.[†]

In examining history and my own karma, as well as the Akashic Record,[‡] I found that the practical and spiri-tual foundations of this spiritual translocation originated in China around 5,000 years ago. This book is about that beginning, and about my part in this process.

Are Thoresen
September 2020

---

* Pulse diagnosis is a very old method of diagnosing diseases, having been used in China for thousands of years. This method may seem in-credible, nonsensical or fraudulent to the Western scientific mind. How-ever, in skilled hands it is a powerful diagnostic method.

† For my full discussion of translocation, see my book *Spiritual Transloca-tion*, Temple Lodge 2020.

‡ The Akashic Record or Chronicle is a compendium of all human events, thoughts, words, emotions and intent ever to have occurred in the past, present, or future. It exists in a non-physical, etheric plane of existence.

Preface

This book is written from my memory of the time I lived in China – a past life or incarnation – 4,000 years ago. I started to write based on only a few memories, but as the writing developed, more and more came to me from the cosmic void of the Akashic Record.

This recovering of memory seems to be an ongoing process, and as more details and memories enable me to fill out the missing parts of the text, further editions of this book may well be published.

Nothing of what is written here can be proved in conventional scientific terms, but for me it is a truth – a clear remembrance and guideline in my ongoing work to relieve the world from the curse of the translocation of disease.

I have several times been directed to my incarnation in China, around 4,000 years ago, working at the royal court of the emperor as a doctor of medicine. This work, as well as the court itself, was for many hundreds of years strongly influenced by the legendary so-called Yellow Emperor,* who ruled China some 1,000 years before I came to dwell in that region.

The first person who directed me to this incarnation was a German colleague, who told me about my incarnation in ancient China as one of the head physicians at

---

* Wikipedia describes him as follows: The Yellow Emperor, also known as the Yellow Thearch, or by his Chinese name Huangdi, is a deity (*shen*) in Chinese religion, one of the legendary Chinese sovereigns and 'culture heroes' included among the mytho-historical Three Sovereigns and Five Emperors and cosmological Five Forms of the Highest Deity.

the court of the emperor. At that time I had apparently misused my magical powers as a healer, and because of this misuse certain celestial forces had taken my healing powers away, leaving me in darkness. In this – my present – incarnation I had finally chosen the right path, and the healing forces had been given back, partly to me and partly to my daughter.

All this is described in detail in the first part of my book *The Forgotten Mysteries of Atlantis,* although in that book only vague mention is made of my incarnation as a physician at the royal court in China.

In the present book, I will first describe how this incarnation in China has influenced my work as a veterinarian in modern-day Norway, and how I was brought to a deeper remembrance of this fatal Chinese experience.

As mentioned already, in my current daily practice as a veterinarian I observed quite early on in my career that all treatments conducted by either orthodox medicine or alternative medicine – especially alternative medicine based on traditional Chinese medicine – caused a *translocation* of disease. That means that the deeper cause of the disease was transferred to other human beings or to animals, and was not really healed or transformed.

I soon began to understand – actually to remember – that the possibility for this to happen was due to some important changes in the philosophical system and practice of medicine made by the Yellow Emperor himself. These changes were refined and developed in the following years by his successors and the leading physicians of his court – through all of whom the Yellow Emperor himself worked spiritually. This included me, and that worried me immensely. What should I do with this knowledge?

The next person who directed me to my Chinese incarnation was also a German (Thomas Mayer), who specializes in reading the Akashic Record when meeting people. While I was explaining the function of the translocation of diseases to a group of Rudolf Steiner's followers in Berlin (I had still not revealed anything about my part in all of this), he told me afterwards that I myself had been a central person in developing the foundations of translocation at the court of one of the Chinese emperors around 4,000 years ago.

This book will deal with that fateful incarnation, some 2,000 years before the incarnation of the Christ – the future redeemer of the ill deeds initiated by the Yellow Emperor. I am writing out of the needs I see at the present time, in order to undo what I did through my professional work some 4,000 years ago.

At that time I was working with 'forging' and 'distorting' of the twelve elements into five elements,* and the changing of the positions of pulse-diagnosis, which made translocation possible. Also, I was partly responsible for the hiding and concealing of knowledge about the possibility for diseases to *transform* and not just translocate – a knowledge that urgently needs to be revealed at the present time.

I see the results of this past work as devastating to contemporary medicine. I see diseases being *translocated* to others, humans or animals, despite the good

---

* A fivefold conceptual scheme that many traditional Chinese fields used to explain a wide array of phenomena, from cosmic cycles to the interaction between internal organs, and from the succession of political regimes to the properties of medicinal drugs. The elements referred to are Fire, Earth, Metal, Water and Wood. More about the fivefold and twelvefold elements will be described in the Introduction.

intentions of many therapists or doctors. I write this as an acceptance of my responsibility for the deeds I performed under the rule of that Chinese emperor.

As we will see from this book, those deeds were actually performed under the rulership of the Yellow Emperor himself – his eternal spirit – working through his successors for several hundred years.

In addition to what in this book is described as the *luciferic force*, there are today two additional adversarial forces that are becoming ever more active: the *ahrimanic* force and the *asuric* force. Both of these forces cooperate with the luciferic force in order to blindfold humanity and lead us astray. But that is the subject for another book.

The Dynasties of China

The Yellow Emperor himself incarnated around 3,000 years before Christ incarnated into the body of Jesus of Nazareth. He is recorded in the ancient texts approximately 2500-3000 BC, where he was first described as the 'God of Light'. Historians falsely claim that he was the first ruler of the Shang Dynasty, derived from Shangdi,* who was considered the highest God of the later Shang Dynasty. Xia Dynasty (2,100 BC – 1,766 BC) was the first dynasty following the incarnation of the

---

"The name Shangdi should be translated as "Highest Deity", but also has the implied meaning of "Primordial Deity" or "First Deity" in Classical Chinese. The deity preceded the title and the emperors of China were named after him in their role as *Tianzi*, the sons of Heaven. In the classical texts the highest conception of the heavens is frequently identified with Shang Di, who is described somewhat anthropomorphically. He is also associated with the pole star. The conceptions of the Supreme ruler (Shang Di) and of the Sublime Heavens (Huang-t'ien) afterward coalesce or absorb each other'. (Wikipedia)

Yellow Emperor. This dynasty is currently considered as 'semi-mythological'. According to the historian Sima Qian in his *Historical Memories*, the Xia dynasty had seventeen kings.

According to the accounts, the last king, Xia Jié, was a tyrant who oppressed and enslaved his people, which precipitated the dynastic change.

Shang Dynasty (1766 BC–1047 BC) is the first dynasty that modern historians can confirm to have existed, due to important archaeological sites found in the Yellow River Valley. Its capital was in Anyang, and its people knew the metallurgy of bronze and techniques of jewellery and armoury. It was a highly hierarchical society, with slaves, soldiers, aristocrats and priests. At the top of the pyramid was King Shang.

This dynasty stood out for its warmongering. Hundreds of Shang graves with dozens of weapons have been found and there is also evidence of human sacrifice. The most famous figure of that period is Fu Hao, a warrior queen or princess.

The dynasties that followed, taking us up to the modern age, were:

- Zhou Dynasty (1047 BC–256 BC)
- Qin Dynasty (221 BC–206 BC)
- Han Dynasty (206 BC–220 AD)
- Three Kingdoms (220–265)
- Jin Dynasty (265–420)
- Southern and Northern Dynasties (386–589)
- Sui Dynasty (581–618)
- Tang Dynasty (618–906)
- Five Dynasties and Ten Kingdoms (907–960)

- Liao Dynasty (907–1125)
- Song Dynasty (960–1279)
- Yuan Dynasty (1279–1368)
- Ming Dynasty (1368–1644)
- Qing Dynasty (1644–1911)

Introduction

The Atlantean heritage. Knowledge of black magic

Thousands of years ago, when the Ice Age was ending in Northern Europe, China was experiencing a period of high spiritual culture. Parallel with the ending of the Ice Age, the Atlantean period and culture also came to an end. Many groups of people fled the threefold destruction of this pre-historic continent, bringing their ancient wisdom to their new homelands.

In Atlantis the totality of knowledge was divided between different groups and different oracles; some of which knew a lot and some of which knew very little. Some groups were characterised by good and constructive wisdom whilst some were dark and destructive (Edgar Cayce* calls the latter groups 'The Sons of Belial'). The differences were marked.

The different groups escaped to different parts of the world, mainly around the Atlantic Ocean.

The groups that fled to America brought to the indigenous American people parts of the spiritual wisdom which also contained the knowledge of the dark or black magic of Atlantis that had finally destroyed that continent. This dark knowledge was developed further under the influence of the strong electric- and

---

* Edgar Cayce (1877-1945) has been called the 'sleeping prophet', the 'father of holistic medicine' and the most documented psychic of the twentieth century. For more than 40 years of his adult life, Cayce gave psychic 'readings' to thousands of seekers whilst in an unconscious state, diagnosing illnesses and revealing lives lived in the past and prophecies yet to come. (from www.edgarcayce.org)

earth-magnetic forces available in America – forces that nourish the ahrimanic powers* in the human body, as for example the doppelgänger. (This black magic reached its peak in Central America under the terrible rule of the Mexican mysteries, described by Rudolf Steiner[†] – see his lecture of 24 September 1916 in his Collected Works, Vol. 171.)

These groups carried within them the magic knowledge of the ahrimanic forces.

The groups that fled to Europe brought different kinds of knowledge, resulting in the different mysteries to be found there during the early period of European culture, in what we today call the Stone Age.

The most important group of all, who had the most complete knowledge – called by Edgar Cayce 'The Sons of the Law of One', and by Rudolf Steiner as 'the highest Sun Initiates' – fled to a place in Central Siberia, from where impulses radiated to all cultures that followed. The seeds of development were thus sown for the cultures that included the Indian, Persian, Egyptian, Greek and, finally, our own period.

This 'Siberian' group – who had full knowledge of the Sun and as such also knowledge of the coming Christ – was the only group that could point to the future.[‡]

---

* See a description of the ahrimanic forces on the next pages.

† Rudolf Joseph Lorenz Steiner (1861–1925) was an Austrian philosopher, author, social reformer, architect and esotericist. He gained initial recognition at the end of the nineteenth century as a literary critic and published philosophical works including *The Philosophy of Freedom*. At the beginning of the twentieth century, he founded an esoteric spiritual movement, anthroposophy, with roots in German idealist philosophy and theosophy.

‡The future as seen as a development in a linear time-concept, and not a cyclic time-concept.

One group, with extensive knowledge of all of the luciferic* cultural light, fled to China. This knowledge was among the most advanced of the time, but it lacked the insight – or at least the acceptance – of the coming Sun impulse, the knowledge that one day the 'Sun emperor' would come to earth and be born to a virgin. Instead, the group honoured and worshipped luciferic knowledge and light. Around 2500-3000 BC, the being of Lucifer himself was able to incarnate within this civilization as the legendary Yellow Emperor, Huangdi.

The Yellow Emperor, Huangdi

Around 3,000 years before Christ and 500-1,000 years before the incarnation of the Yellow Emperor, an event of huge importance occurred. During this event the whole world experienced something strange and fatal. During only a period of a few weeks, the whole spiritual world seemed to disappear for every single person in the world. People still spoke about this during my incarnation 1,000 years later.

The disappearance of the spiritual world started with a deep sleep that came over all human beings. This sleep lasted for three weeks. Thousands did not survive that sleep, and the number of living human beings was drastically reduced. After that we all lived in spiritual darkness. The wise ones said that the whole cosmos had entered the dark age, the *Kali Yuga*.

Five hundred years after this fatal event, 2,500 years before Christ, a powerful wizard came from the northwest, from what today we call the Gobi Desert, an area

---

* See a description of the luciferic forces on the following pages.

south-east of where the 'Siberian group' lingered. He emerged out of this spiritual darkness, and was – due to his immense spiritual powers – immediately accepted as the 'ruler'. He brought both light and a great and immense knowledge of mass-psychology and warfare, and soon he was able to gather a large number of smaller clans under his rulership. This emperor was called Huangdi, and this name later gave rise to the Xia Dynasty (2100 BC–1766 BC). Huangdi was originally an unnamed being, only referred to as 'the Lord of the Underworld', and was usually depicted as or with a dragon. His mother, Fubao, was according to legend a virgin who, through an immaculate conception, conceived him after being hit by a bolt of lightning.

Who are Lucifer and Ahriman?

As the being of Lucifer – and his counterpart Ahriman – are integral to this book, we will see how Rudolf Steiner characterized these beings and those that serve them. In a lecture he held on 21 November 1919, he states:

> We may say that we picture the outward characteristics of luciferic beings properly when we imagine that they possess such forces as we human beings manifest when we become visionaries, when we abandon ourselves one-sidedly to fantasy, let ourselves be carried away, and, speaking metaphorically, lose our heads. In other words, whenever we tend to go out beyond our heads, we are dealing with forces that, while they play a certain role in our organism, actually belong cosmically to the beings we term luciferic. If we imagine beings who are

wholly formed of that tendency in us that strives to
go out beyond our heads, we are picturing the luciferic beings who are related to our human world in
certain ways.

Now, in contrast, think of everything that presses
us down upon the earth, that makes us dull and
philistine, leading us to develop materialistic atti-
tudes, penetrating us with a dry intellect, and so on:
there you have a picture of ahrimanic powers.

He adds:

We may characterize these two kinds of beings still
further. For instance, we may contemplate luciferic
beings in terms of the kind of interest they take in
cosmic existence. We find that their chief interest
lies in making the world, particularly the human
world, unfaithful to the spiritual beings whom we
must regard as the true creators of humanity. Their
one desire is to make the world disloyal to these
divine beings. They are not interested in claiming
the world for themselves. You will have gathered
from previous remarks about luciferic beings that
that is not their chief aim. Their aim is rather to
make human beings forsake their divine creator-be-
ings – they wish to free the world from the beings
felt by humankind to be the real divinities.

The ahrimanic beings have a different interest.
Their firm intention is to get the human kingdom
and thereby the earth along with it into their sphere
of power, to make human beings dependent on
them, to control humanity. Whereas luciferic beings
strive, and have always striven, to alienate us from
the beings whom we feel to be our Gods, ahrimanic

beings seek to draw humanity and everything connected with it into their power.

In other words, luciferic beings striving for universal freedom, and ahrimanic beings striving for lasting dominion, are constantly waging war in this cosmos we are part of.[*]

In the same lecture, Rudolf Steiner speaks of a cosmic 'triad':

Contemplating all this, you will notice that the world can really be understood only in terms of a triad. On one side we have everything luciferic, on the other everything ahrimanic, and, in the third, central, place, the point of balance between the two, humanity, with a sense of its relationship to the divine, of its divine essence. We can understand the world in the right way only when we see it based on this triad and are perfectly clear that human life is the beam of the scales. Here is the fulcrum: on one side is the luciferic element, actually pulling the pan upwards; opposite is the ahrimanic element, pushing the pan downwards. Our human task – our human essence – is to keep the beam balanced.

But humanity is not alone in this task. We are supported by the being of Christ, who we know incarnated on earth two thousand years ago as Jesus Christ. However, Steiner also speaks of both Lucifer and Ahriman incarnating on earth. Steiner's premise is that Ahriman will incarnate in the West, before 'a part' of this third millennium has passed – as a counterpoint to the physical incarnation of Lucifer in the East in the third millennium BC. The

---

[*] See Rudolf Steiner, *The Incarnation of Ahriman*, Rudolf Steiner Press 2006.

balancing point is the incarnation at the beginning of the modern era of Jesus Christ in Palestine, whose culminating deed Steiner calls the 'Mystery of Golgotha'.

*

Rudolf Steiner recounts the beginning of our evolution by reminding us that our human soul contained, from the beginning, a powerful primeval wisdom. But in the beginning the seed of this wisdom had to be nurtured to achieve the spiritual heights we needed to attain to become developed beings in material existence. We needed a spiritual guide from the higher hierarchies to assist us in the growth of our 'I'-consciousness. This teacher was the descended archangel called Lucifer.

Chinese Thought and Philosophy before the Yellow Emperor

The following is technical, and perhaps mainly relevant to alternative medical practitioners. However, it is important background to the story of my past life that I tell in the following chapters.

For hundreds or maybe thousands of years before the Yellow Emperor changed the medical system in 3000 BC, the Chinese had a twelve-element system, based on the twelve streams of etheric energy streaming down from the zodiac – or rather from the area behind the zodiacal signs. In this system, man and woman (Yin and Yang) were separate and worked independently.

In changing the twelvefold world perception into a five-element one, the main difference was that Yin and Yang were put together within the same element: Liver with Gall bladder in the Wood element, Kidney with Bladder in the Water element, Spleen with Stomach in the Earth element, Lung with Large intestine in the Metal element, Pericardium with Triple Heater in the Fire element and also Heart with Small intestine in the Fire element. We see here also that 'Warmth' and 'Fire', represented by the Heart and the Sexual Organs were put together as Heart and Pericardium, both within the Fire element. Thus, the differences between sex and love and between fire and warmth were confused, which today benefits highly both the luciferic and ahrimanic forces.

This resulted in both man and woman – as well as love and sex – being perceived as merged together, their differences concealed. According to Dr Johannes Weinzirl, one of the leaders of anthroposophic medical education, this is a main cause of diseases being transferred from parents to children.

This confusion also happened in European culture in the 1970s, when the differences between man and woman, between sex and love, were obscured, and resulted in massive waves of translocated diseases, such as cancer.

The same deceit took place in the pulse diagnostic system. Before the time of the Yellow Emperor, the positions of Yin and Yang, male and female, were far apart – actually diametrically so. Now they were put together at the wrist of the human being, bringing man and woman together as if they were the same – as if they were one – thus preparing for the possibility of translocation.

Interestingly enough, the five-element system paved the way for an easier translocation of the luciferic part of the symptom-complex, but not the ahrimanic part.

As the Yellow Emperor was of a luciferic nature – and actually was Lucifer himself (as will later become apparent) – his system and thinking facilitated the survival of his own legions of demons. In this way, he looks after his own servants.

Why the Yellow Emperor was, and always will be, a Myth

Today, and also in the period following the rule of the Yellow Emperor, many people thought that the 'Yellow God' was a mythical figure. The reason for this was that very few people really knew who he was. The Yellow Emperor was in reality the *spirit* embodying the ruler, and as he usually spoke and worked through many of the dominating men within the court, it was often difficult to know exactly who he was.

Sometimes the spirit of the Yellow Emperor spoke and acted through my own father in that incarnation. I witnessed this once in my fifteenth year. At this time, several systems of pulse diagnosis were in operation, and a meeting between the most influential doctors was held in the emperor's palace. When my father was asked to speak, his visage changed completely. He became strong and a certain powerful energy radiated from his very being and in every word he uttered. In that moment his importance became so great that everybody listened, and his views became a foundation for the development of pulse diagnosis. Before then several systems were used, but afterwards only one system became standard. This system brought Yin and Yang together at the wrists, and man and woman were thus addressed together. The only difference between them was that a slightly stronger pressure was used to read women's energies than when reading those of men.

The real spirit of the 'Yellow God' thus overshadowed all of the men in power, and especially when they were in a significant situation. Then they could utter words that the Yellow God wanted, and he spoke through them. Of course, he mostly spoke through the ruler, the emperor. In this way, most people at the court were uncertain who their emperor really was.

Chapter One

*Life at the court of the Chinese emperor Yu the Great
(c. 2123–2025 BC), in the pre-dynastic time leading up to the
Xia dynasty*

Being a physician at the Chinese court of the pre-dynastic emperor 4,000 years ago was a life of constant anxiety, being both watchful of your enemies and fearful for your own life.

This work was usually inherited from father to son, and I was born into such a lineage. My father was a royal physician, a highly esteemed doctor of the court, and he had a wealth of secret knowledge relating to both white and black magic. Indeed, his knowledge was mainly magical, concerning the creation and healing of diseases, as well as the differences between transformation and translocation of pathological demonic forces to other people or to animals.

At that time everybody knew very well that all diseases were due to and dependent upon the existence of adversarial or demonic forces. A good doctor could weaken or strengthen such demons, and would either transform them within the patient or translocate them to another human being or animal.

A person who could master this technique could be very dangerous, and as my father had such knowledge in abundance, this led to and caused him to be killed when I was 25-years-old, in an official execution that we all had to witness.

However, by the time of his death, my father had already transmitted to me everything he knew. This teaching was especially related to influencing the spirits that caused disease, but also spirits that 'stimulated' spirituality. Many spirits opened portals to the spiritual world and lived in different more-or-less poisonous plants – plants that today are used in the same way, but are now classified as drugs or psychedelics.

My father's knowledge related to how to influence or modify these spirits by means of different plants, vibrations, acupuncture points and the use of various metals.

My father was offered the 'honourable possibility' of committing suicide, which at that time was somehow considered better that being beheaded, but he refrained from this, knowing full well that, having worked with black magic, a suicide would be detrimental to his karma. Suicide would have caused his black deeds to boomerang back to him, whereas being killed by others would have enabled him to work with his karma in a much more effective way.

The emperor also knew this very well, and this was one of the reasons why my father was executed, as he had become too powerful. The emperor *wanted* him to commit suicide, and eventually he succeeded in his wish as my father was betrayed. The character of the betrayal was that he was tricked into committing suicide. Before the beheading he was offered a glass of bitter water as a sedative and painkiller. He was made to believe that the water contained an extract of opium. This tincture tastes quite bitter. However, it was not opium but an extract of bitter almonds, and not knowing that the water was poisoned he drank it, thus dying by his own hand.

This was the lesser part of the betrayal, and it partly caused the black deeds to be thrown back upon himself. The worst part of the betrayal was the kind of poison that was used, and how this poison then worked on my father's memory in the time between death and rebirth and especially in his next life.

An extract of bitter almonds works in a very special way on the reflecting abilities of the etheric body. This reflecting in the etheric world is the only possibility we have to realize our mistakes after death, and is the foundation of the meeting of the so-called Guardian of the Threshold or the Animals of the Abyss. Without being able to see ourselves after death as a reflection in the etheric world, as both a likeness and an image, we have great difficulties in transforming our darker deeds as a preparation for our next life. But when our deeds of black magic are cast back on us as well, the situation becomes extremely difficult.

When taken voluntarily, this bitter almond extract thus works on the etheric memory in a destructive way. The poison splinters the etheric memory-mirror, just like a physical mirror is splintered, and the unchanged deeds of black magic are thrown back upon one in a way that is very frightening.

Memory of the etheric forces is stored in the spiritual world, and a human being's mind is able to reflect the part of this memory that he has made conscious. In this way we can remember everything that we have made conscious. But an extract from bitter almonds splinters this mirror, so that after death we cannot transform anything.

The emperor did not want my father ever again – in any future life – to challenge his power. In this way, he wanted to get rid of all kinds of competition for ever, in all future incarnations!

I avoided this deceit when I was also murdered some twenty-five years later. I will describe this later. I will also explain how I was able to lift the twofold curse from my father's shoulders, about two years after his death – the curse that the Yellow Emperor had so brutally and covertly caused him to suffer.

*

One of the usual excuses to execute a leading Chinese doctor at the court of the emperor— actually any royal healer or physician—was not that he had become too powerful or too clever, but that he had failed to cure a member of the royal family or another very important person.

At that time, as in all ancient cultures, all diseases were experienced as having a spiritual background. It is actually only in our Western culture, during the last 250 years, that diseases are considered to have non-spiritual origins. Today diseases are considered 'accidental' and having very little to do with what we do, think, feel or behave – and the healing of diseases is believed to depend on the medicines given and our natural healing powers, not the spiritual insights and power of the healer or doctor. The spiritual view of disease is today mostly held only by some anthroposophic doctors, new-age practitioners or within certain shamanistic traditions.

The failure to heal a disease 4,000 years ago meant that the doctor had no spiritual power, and was therefore 'expendable'. All diseases were considered to be related to the presence of spirits or demonic powers, and the healing of them was considered to be highly depen-dent on the spiritual powers and insights of the doctor or healer.

Most if not all 'healing' of sick people (from 3,000 years BC until today) was actually due to the fact that the pathological demons creating the symptoms were translocated to another entity – a person, animal, tree, or plant.

For the men in power, other than translocating all pathology to others, the most important thing was to keep themselves healthy by preventing the transloca-tion of the demonic entities that caused disease to them-selves. To avoid this, it was important to sustain a high level of Qi energy. The pathological demons need an open space in order to be able to 'infect' a person; they need a void into which they can enter. Therefore, these healers tried to build up their internal energy and not waste it through hard work, worries or too much sex.*

There were different methods to build up Qi energy, which are still valid today. Qi is received through:

- Food, spices and water via the digestive system.
- Air and smells via the lungs and the skin.
- Vibrational energy through all twelve sense-or-gans, especially the eyes, ears, nose, touch and taste (a kiss for example is very energy-giving).
- A final way was to take different kinds of energy from other living entities, almost like a sort of vampirism. Such sources could be:
  - plants and trees;
  - animals;

---

*Today an additional method is to develop a strong 'I'-consciousness, especially one that has allowed the Christ-force into one's heart.

- ◦ other human beings, especially:
  - • women, as female energy is very satisfying to powerful men;
  - • children, as their energy is seldom imbued with 'I'-consciousness, and can easily be misused for dark deeds. (It goes without saying that this was – and still is – an abhorrent practice.)

Female energy was considered especially beneficial for most men, especially from young women – and even, tragically, from girls. The use of young women and children to keep men in general – especially men in higher positions such as the emperor* – 'filled with energy' was very well known within this culture.

In my Atlantean incarnation as an oracle, I frequently extracted great amounts of energy from other human beings through violent methods. These practices could not be used after the Great Flood that destroyed the Atlantean continent, and also destroyed certain powers that previously made it possible to utilize energy in this aggressive way. Therefore, within the Chinese culture of that time, such 'vampirism' had to be conducted in other ways.

For several incarnations after that Chinese one, I utilized consciously or unconsciously these 'new' methods

---

* It seems that this knowledge and practice is still in use today among the powerful – and royalty – of modern-day high society. See for example Mick Jagger, who has fathered eight children from five different women, of whom it has been said: 'I think he's like a sex vampire. Being with all these different people makes him feel young and gives him all this energy.' (Natasha Terry speaking in *The Daily Mail*, 16 July 2012.) (See also the Jeffrey Epstein or Harvey Weinstein cases – or even the allegations against a member of the British Royal Family – Editor.)

of taking female energy.* We can see this practice today, especially in the 'left-hand' brotherhoods – i.e. in all groups that practice black magic. To observe how energy is harvested and gathered in special ways is one of the crucial 'signs' as to whether a group is of the 'right-' or 'left-hand' tradition.†

The emperor had for this purpose also many women, young girls and children at his disposal – females that did not mean anything to him, but were kept merely as sources of 'energy'.‡

I will describe this female energy in further detail. It is different from the energy of the cosmos or nature. From all areas of the cosmos, from the planetary realm, from the stellar (zodiacal) realm and also from the vast void behind the stellar area, as well as from the natural world, enormous amounts of etheric§ energy can be received or harvested. This can be used for many purposes, such as bestowing long life, health, physical power and also

---

* This is described in Part III of my book *The Forgotten Mysteries of Atlantis.*

† Societies that practice black or white magic are called 'left-hand' or 'right-hand' brotherhoods respectively

‡ These women were treated as 'batteries', just as described in the film *The Matrix.*

§ Etheric energy is the energy that supports life – the energy that our growing, thinking and life forces depend upon. This etheric energy streams through all aspects of the cosmos, including the great illusion of the material world and the semi illusion of the three realms of the elemental world, where the etheric energy expresses itself in elemental beings. There are four forms of this etheric energy: 1/ life-ether that expresses itself in gnomes; 2/ chemical ether that expresses itself in the undines; 3/ light ether that expresses itself in the sylphs; and 4/ warmth ether that expresses itself in the salamanders. It also exists within the twelve celestial pastel colour streams within the etheric world itself – the pure world behind the elemental world.

magic. In the future this kind of energy can and will be used also for white magic, i.e. for the 'three occult-isms' that Rudolf Steiner speaks of: 'hygienic occultism' in healing diseases, 'mechanical occultism' in working machines, driving cars or flying planes (which will at some point replace electricity), and in 'eugenic occult-ism', in regulating and deciding where and when birth and death are to take place.

This etheric energy can in general be received either directly, semi-directly or indirectly, and the differences here are of crucial importance.

- The direct stream can only be used for good, i.e. for white magic.
- The semi-direct stream, via the sexual organs, can be used for both good and evil, although it is usually used for darker purposes.
- The indirect stream, via the earth, can only be used for darker or black magic.

The direct energy comes straight from plants, trees and animals, from other humans, the planets, or the wide expanses of the cosmos behind the zodiac.

The indirect way comes about when this energy pene-trates the earth and is then mirrored back into the body, thus changed by the adversarial forces inhabiting the earth. These earth-forces are mainly demonic and of an ahrimanic type.

There is also a middle way, a semi-direct stream, apart from the direct and the earth-related streams, and that is the sexual stream. Energy that is used in this way does not penetrate the earth, but goes in through the lower parts of the human being, often the sexual organs, and from here streams up into the rest of the body. This energy can be used for both white and black magic, but – as mentioned above – mainly has the potential for black magic.

The first kind (the direct stream) works spiritually in an up-building way, the second (the indirect one) works in an ahrimanic, destructive way. The third stream, from the lower human parts, can be used in both ways. However, if the receiver doesn't realize where the energy has come from, all three streams can feel as if they have great potency and beneficial effect.

- The energy from nature can be received both directly and indirectly, but seldom as the semi-direct, sexual stream. The direct stream is spiritual and the indirect form, which passes through the earth before entering the human body, is ahrimanic. The semi-direct stream is partly luciferic, partly ahrimanic and partly 'white'.

- We can also receive energy from animals, again in two ways – directly or via the dark forces of the earth, as with the third stream. The semi-direct stream is again seldom used, although in rare cases this may happen, but is considered an abnormality. The direct stream of energy from animals, at least from higher animals,* communicates with human energy through the animals' group-soul. This exchange happens in the upper layers of the atmosphere called the thermosphere, ninety kilometres above the earth, where

---

*I will not elaborate here on the lower forms or insects.

the Northern Lights occur.* From there it can enter humans directly or indirectly, as described above. The indirect stream relates to the slaughter of animals – the letting of blood – and is reflected in the rules of 'halal'.

- The energy coming from female groups or single individuals dedicated or bound to a male, can theoretically enter the man's energetic body in all three ways. In ancient times this was true, but after the incarnation of Christ the indirect way via the earth is almost impossible. So, today only the direct and the semi-direct are possible. Although these three streams can originate from the same individual and as such have the same character, in my experience they are still like three different types.

Female Energy

The following is based on spiritual-scientific observation, and is meant in general terms – not as creating stereotypes.

Women in general have a much bigger and wider etheric body than men. This goes for their astral body as well. Women also give away their energy quite freely; they care for the world around them as if they are duty-bound to nourish the whole world. Men are much more restricted in the way they hold both their etheric and astral energy for themselves. In this way, they are much

---

* The Sámi children are taught to be afraid of the animal energy coming from or through the Northern Lights, as they can become 'crazy' when animal energy enters them, both directly or indirectly. They are told to hide in the snow when the Northern Lights come too close.

more egoistic than women regarding the use of their energy.

As mentioned, many men and even some women feed on the energy from other human beings – especially from women – in a kind of vampirism. This especially goes for men in power, such as politicians, musicians, religious leaders and gurus.

The energetic stream that women can give to other beings, especially men in power – and of course to children – leaves their bodies mainly through the lower chakras, but is received differently by men, either directly, semi-directly or indirectly. The importance of how to receive this energy has changed over the millennia, and is quite different today than what it was in ancient Atlantis.

How the Energy coming from Women can be 'Harvested' by Men

To reiterate and expand on what was said earlier:

The direct stream comes through the upper part—the head or the sense organs—and then streams down into the body, through all the organs, building them up in a good and constructive way. This stream follows the blood vessels, thus connecting it to the family bloodstream. This stream resembles the described direct stream from the cosmos or nature. This energy cannot be misused, in dark magical ways, in order to obtain power.

The semi-direct stream goes directly to the lower part of the body, to the area of the sexual organs – even a little down into the earth – and from there streams up through the nervous system. The peculiarity of this stream, this special kind of energy, is that it can also influence the bloodstream. It is thus not only semi-direct but semi-functional. It can affect both the blood and the nervous system, and for those that can wield this kind of energy, it has a very multi-potent ability. With people who use black magic, this kind of energy is highly valued. Stories of medieval black magicians who harvest energy by means of sexual rites have their origin in this knowledge.

The indirect stream goes first into the earth, often quite deeply, and then streams up through the body. This energy, that has been in contact with the ahrimanic forces of the earth, automatically seeks its way through the nerves, as ahrimanic forces dominate the nerves. This stream is negative, full of power and can be used to perform all kinds of darker magic.

This last kind of energy, the indirect stream, I myself used during my incarnation in Atlantis, thousands of years ago, and this energy made me capable of performing the dark deeds I was responsible for. The 'harvesting' done in Atlantis was, though, of a totally different kind to the 'harvesting' done 4,000 years ago – and still different to how it is done today.

The energy could be harvested indirectly 20,000 years ago. This was difficult 4,000 years ago, and today it is impossible.

Types of Energy Harvesting

In old Atlantis: The energy from humans, especially from women, was harvested by use of black magic, using a magical 'tie' that hindered the 'thinking energy' from mingling with the heart—'feeling energy'; and then both thinking energy and feeling energy could be 'taken' separately and used for different purposes. This stolen energy could then be absorbed, both through the direct stream and via the indirect or semi-direct way – it did not matter how. The 'giver' of energy had no influence as to how the energy was used.

In China 4,000 years ago: At this time the energy was harvested by exerting full dominion over women or young girls, usually by direct tapping from the lower chakras. The absorption of the energy could now either be through the direct, semi-direct or indirect way, and this also decided their use. The energy-giver again had little influence over how the energy was used by the man who was 'harvesting' it.

Today: Gathering energy from women is usually done in secrecy or subconsciously – in some cases consciously – by first establishing a 'guru'-relationship to a woman. Then, the energy that the woman freely gives is taken in either through the direct or the semi-direct path. Today, energy from humans cannot be absorbed via the indirect way, although energy from nature and the cosmos can also still be taken via the indirect way. The quality of the given energy is of crucial importance as to how it can be used. If it is imbued with the 'I'-force of the giver, it can never be used for evil; but if it is void of 'I'-consciousness, it can be used by the harvester as he or she wishes.

Today the direct stream is imbued with consciousness, with understanding, with the 'I'-conscious power of the giver, and this energy gives rise to good deeds – to a constructive building up of the body and an ability to perform good deeds.

The other stream, the semi-direct, is darker, both because it is related to the lower chakras, to lack of 'I'-consciousness of the 'giver', and to sexual desire, and as such connected to both luciferic and ahrimanic forces.

The lack of 'I'-consciousness comes when girls or young women lack understanding with their conscious minds. This is why today their energy is sought by those wanting to use it for egotistic power and darker deeds, as they have less 'I'-consciousness than adult or mature women.

This unconscious energy was what the Chinese emperor and the men at his court liked best.

Chapter Two

Failings and executions

My father was one of the most valued physicians at the royal court. He was given great respect and had almost unlimited power. His every command had to be followed by the women, soldiers, servants and slaves.

He also had the ability to command many kinds of adversarial spirits, especially luciferic ones. In this way he could easily observe the luciferic spirits causing diseases, both physical and mental. He knew how to transform these spirits, something which the emperor had forbidden as he did not want them to be transformed. They were considered holy and untouchable.

In earlier times, a transformation of the luciferic and ahrimanic spirits was possible due to the strong magical force of the initiates of the Mysteries. This power had been lost by 3100 BC, by which time the clairvoyant forces had left humanity, except in a few cases. When the world entered the period of *Kali Yuga*, and we were all left in spiritual darkness, our ability to *transform* was also lost. It was not until the coming of the Christ that such a transformation was once again possible, but then in a completely different manner: not through force, but with grace.

However, as the transforming force of Christ was then still in the distant future, it was quite difficult to transform these luciferic spirits. This was the time of the luciferic forces and spirits – between 3100 BC and 1500 AD – and they were not to be touched. After that came the time of the ahrimanic spirits, but that will be described in a future book.

The luciferic spirits were causing a lot of disease, and if such diseases attached to people in power—the royals and the wealthy—something had to be done. Therefore, the spirits had to be translocated to people at a lower level in society, who were, so to speak, sacrificed in honour of the luciferic force. Everyone accepted this, in all old cultures, including the Jewish one.

This is the reason why blood sacrifice was so widely used and accepted as a deed of necessity in almost all cultures of the pre-Christian age. Blood sacrifice of animals was actually one of the most common methods to translocate diseases. The luciferic disease was transferred into the animal by the force and insight of the priest, and then the demon was translocated further when blood was shed. This blood was then washed away by huge amounts of water, often into a pool or lake, such as Bethesda (in Jerusalem).

Let us now describe this procedure – although in this story the demons took the path via swine and into water. The Bible tells the tale of a man who was sick from a multiplicity of demons, named *Legio* or Legion. When Jesus arrived, the demons begged him to let them go into a herd of swine nearby, probably because they did not want to be transformed. Jesus allowed them this, and the *Legio* of demons flew into the pig herd. The swine went crazy, fled into the water and drowned,* washed away by the water.

---

* Luke 8:26: 'Then they sailed to the country of the Gerasenes, which is opposite Galilee. 27 And when He came out onto the land, He was met by a man from the city who was possessed with demons; and who had not put on any clothing for a long time, and was not living in a house, but in the tombs. 28 Seeing Jesus, he cried out and fell before Him, and said in a loud voice, "What business do we have with each other, Jesus,

From my father I learned how to translocate any form of disease. I was taught different procedures to translocate the demons: through blood-letting of the patient (even to the point of death); through translocation via the blood of an animal; through magic rites or verses, or through acupuncture or herbs.

But seldom or never was the possibility of a *transformation* discussed – that would be considered a crime towards the emperor himself, as the 'Yellow God' held his protective hand over the luciferic demonic forces that caused disease.

In investigating the differences between translocation and a transformation, I later found out how to lift the twofold curse that – after the deceit and execution of my father – had held him in a magical prison.

Son of the Most High God? I beg You, do not torment me." 29 For He had commanded the unclean spirit to come out of the man. For it had seized him many times; and he was bound with chains and shackles and kept under guard, and yet he would break his bonds and be driven by the demon into the desert. 30 And Jesus asked him, "What is your name?" And he said, "Legion"; for many demons had entered him. 31 They were imploring Him not to command them to go away into the abyss. 32 Now there was a herd of many swine feeding there on the mountain; and the demons implored Him to permit them to enter the swine. And He gave them permission. 33 And the demons came out of the man and entered the swine; and the herd rushed down the steep bank into the lake and was drowned. 34 When the herdsmen saw what had happened, they ran away and reported it in the city and out in the country. 35 The people went out to see what had happened; and they came to Jesus, and found the man from whom the demons had gone out, sitting down at the feet of Jesus, clothed and in his right mind; and they became frightened. 36 Those who had seen it reported to them how the man who was demon-possessed had been made well. 37 And all the people of the country of the Gerasenes and the surrounding district asked Him to leave them, for they were gripped with great fear; and He got into a boat and returned.'

In translocating diseases, the powers of the 'turned around' energy-streams from the earth (described earlier as the indirect energy streams), were used in a black magical way. These are the streams that come from all living things and the cosmos, enter the earth and are then returned, thus coming from the darker forces of the earth itself.

It is also possible to use the non-'I'-conscious streams* coming from women, young females and children in this way. These streams 'power up' both the luciferic and the ahrimanic entities or structures, and always make the adversarial demonic powers stronger. In making them stronger, they can also be translocated or led to other living beings.

In most, if not all, historical or contemporary shamanistic healings, translocations initiated mainly with the help of such forces were and still are used.

Because my father was executed and betrayed by the emperor, I developed a deep resistance to the governing power, and I began, in secret, to investigate the whole area of adversarial demons, how they caused disease, how they were translocated, strengthened or weakened. I learned a lot. I also started to see the possibility of transforming these demonic forces.

During my work I discovered that there was also another kind of energy stream: the stream that came directly from the cosmos, the planets, the void behind the zodiac, from both animals and plants and of course also from 'I'-conscious women or even 'I'-conscious children – although the latter was rare. This energy helped transform the strength of the luciferic and ahrimanic

---

* The nature of these streams is explained in Chapter One.

demonic forces, and it was a discovery that amazed me. I spent a lot of time understanding it.

In working with this energy, I discovered that it could not be used to do evil or to translocate diseases. It could only be used for transformation of diseases and also for other good or moral deeds. I also discovered that such direct energy streams could rebuild an etheric body that had been destroyed by black magic. The good energy was even stronger than the grey or black variants, the semi-direct and the indirect versions of energy.

After the darkening of the spiritual world that happened in 3101 BC, this kind of energy was very difficult to trace or understand. It was as if the whole cosmos had darkened in its spiritual aspect. Still, by deducing what was taught in the emperor's private temple and reading between the lines, I found out that the direct energy that could transform the pathological forces had to do with the forces coming from the cosmos in the evening and in the morning. There were strict rules, given by the emperor, that weapons and medicines were not to be made in the evening or morning, as they would then contain a certain energy that inspired the user to do moral actions, and that did not fit the scheme of war or translocation. Medicines and weapons had to be made in the middle of the day or night.

When I later built up my bodyguard with 'special' soldiers, I had to 'prepare' these soldiers during the midnight hours. This could not be done during the morning and evening hours.

When I began to understand the differences between the direct and good forces and the other two streams, I started to experiment with all three streams. As I already had a lot of knowledge and experience with the semi-direct and indirect streams from the years my father was alive to educate me, my main interest was to explore the effects of the direct stream of energy. I found out that this direct energy could regenerate and change a shattered and destroyed etheric sheath.*

With this knowledge I tried to use this energy to save my father, who was captured in limbo between the earth and the Moon-sphere. I was able to send a strong beam of 'white' energy towards him, and thus I helped him to regain and rebuild his splintered etheric 'mirror'.

I succeeded in this. He had been constantly bombarded with the evil deeds he had done, unable to 'defend' himself as if his hands were bound. He had also been unable to see these deeds clearly, and thus was unable to understand what was going on. The stream of white etheric energy I was able to direct towards him managed to rebuild the splintered mirror and free him, so that after a while he was able both to understand the deeds he had done and also to transform them in a way that made him able to proceed on his way in the afterlife – to proceed through the Moon-sphere, towards the Venus-sphere, the Mercury-sphere and lastly to get to the Sun-sphere. After a long time he was 'saved' by my actions and new insights.

I revealed none of this knowledge to anyone at court. Not, that is, until this incarnation and in this book. Now it is time to reveal these secrets – to divide the energy streams above from those of below, and separate the forces of Yin and Yang in both the five-element circle and the pulse-positions.

This work is described in more detail in my book *Spiritual Translocation*.

---

* In this regard, for practitioners of acupuncture I have written a book entitled *Acupuncture and Translocation*.

Chapter Three

Corruption of the direct forces. The obedience to the luciferic powers and the deceit of true healing

As we have seen, the Chinese culture of that time promoted a medical system that preferred translocation to transformation. This is because:

- The presence of adversarial elemental beings, demons, was obvious to them. Thus, a conscious promotion of either translocation or transformation could be considered.
- Transformation would weaken the luciferic forces (as today it would weaken the ahrimanic forces), and this would in turn weaken the powers of the emperor.
- The mindset of the Chinese culture was to preserve the existing system, and a transformation would threaten this mindset.
- In a strong hierarchical system, the people lower down in the pyramid are considered to be less important. There were no moral implications to inflicting them with disease.
- Transformation would require use of direct etheric forces, and this knowledge would weaken the philosophic system of Chinese culture.
- Transformation would also depend on the use of the morning–evening forces, and the knowledge of these forces was not understood by the Chinese culture of the time.

- As translocation is faster and more effective than transformation, this of course promoted the healers who practiced translocation.
- As transformation is often followed by an aggravation of the symptoms, it demands much more work or energy than translocation; therefore the healers that use the method of translocation are often preferred by patients.
- In today's world, even the thought of translocation would be considered immoral. At that time in China, morality was quite different. The Chinese had, and many still have, a strong belief in karma, just like Indian culture, and if a disease was translocated to anybody, especially someone of the lower classes, it was considered to be the karmic will of the gods, which should therefore be suffered in calm and tranquillity.

From the above points, we can conclude that Chinese doctors preferred translocation. And at this stage of evolution they were not even able or allowed to consider transformation of any disease. Diseases were to be translocated, full stop.

In ancient China, such a translocation depended on the knowledge and insights of the healer, shaman or doctor. Today this is still so, but a true transformation is more dependent on the cosmic Christ-force mediated by the morning–evening forces than the healer's personal powers.

Because such a translocation-based 'healing' depended mostly on the powers and insights of the healer, the ability to heal was attributed to the powers of the doctor in question. If he or she could not heal a disease, that meant that his or her powers were not sufficient to practice as a healer, and that he or she should therefore not be a healer.

The merciless executions of doctors who did not manage to heal disease in an effective way was also an effective promotion of the way the Yellow Emperor and his successors worked, i.e. translocation. Doctors did not dare to even *try* to transform a disease.

The demand the court put to a healer was that he should be able to heal any disease in a very short time, either with herbs, formulas, spells or acupuncture. In this way the most effective methods were preferred.

As it is always easier to translocate a disease than to transform it, translocation-based methods, herbal formulas or acupuncture were preferred. Methods that tried to induce a transformation of the disease always led to more pain, aggravation or work than the translocation-based methods. Also, in transforming a disease the doctor has to point to faults and mistakes in the thinking, feeling and will of the patient, and to do this to royalty was nigh on impossible.

My Secret Experiments with Translocation versus Transformation

My father had been condemned to an eternity of oblivion and, because I had managed to save him, this led to several changes in my outlook:

- I lost my reverence for the absolute power and acceptance of the demi-godlike authority that most people attributed to the emperor.
- I learned to know the three streams of etheric energy. In later lives this led me to understand

both healing powers and the importance of Christ-energy and Christ-consciousness.

- I started to understand how to transform a disease, and also the implications of translocation.

Privately I started to experiment with methods that could transform disease. To do so, I first had to find how to distinguish a translocation from a transformation, which I discovered was very easy:

- The main signs that a disease has been translocated is that the patient immediately feels relieved, as if something has just left them.
- The main sign that a disease has started to transform is that the symptoms start to change, and then the patient feels changed. Often old memories of trauma show up in dreams or in waking consciousness. A deep transformation may take some months to achieve.
- Sometimes the disease just translocates to another organ or to another part of the body. Here, the symptoms usually show themselves quite differently than before, so that the patient believes a different condition is manifesting, which of course it is. But it is still the same demonic structure that had harmed the patient previously.
- If the treatment is strong enough, the pathological entity (usually the luciferic demon) is expelled from the patient's body, and this can be seen as a fog. This fog is not physical of course, it is purely etheric, but can still be seen with the help of a clairvoyant eye.

- A transformation often requires gentle treatment. In this way, many acupuncture treatments, strong herbal mixtures and similar strong stimuli lead to translocation. Soft and careful treatment—only one needle, gentler herbs—leads to a transformation of the disease.

To understand the difference between transforming and translocating healing methods, it might be useful to compare the treatment of young criminals by a 'bad cop' versus a 'good cop' method, or the treatment by a 'soft' parent versus a 'violent' parent. We can imagine which method might make the young criminal run away, and which method might keep him listening, so that in time he might become a law-abiding citizen.

Because of the obvious immediate 'benefits' of the translocative method, the whole system of healing became corrupted. Then, combined with the lack of morality and compassion in the culture of that time, this led to a broad acceptance of the phenomenon of translocation. As long as the patients were happy and nobody knew where the pathological demon went, everything was fine. Thus healing modalities became totally corrupted.

It was also generally accepted and known that the emperor, being in close contact with the 'Yellow God' (which we have referred to as the luciferic deity), did not accept any transforming of the entities causing disease. He only accepted their translocation. A transformation of the luciferic entities would ultimately diminish his own power and strength, and he would not allow this. However, the emperor would not accept that any demon be translocated to himself or to any of his family or friends, or to any other person in power!

This was not a problem however, as pathological demons, entities or demonic energy only translocate to a weaker person or animal – and as all the important and powerful people had numerous ways to 'steal' energy from servants, women and children, the diseases seldom found their way to affecting these dignitaries.

Personal Experiments with Transformation and Translocation

My experiments with trying to influence spirits responsible for disease and spirituality were done mainly after and in connection with my work to save my father from his double spiritual imprisonment.

I experimented with:

- *The three streams* – these investigations were of the utmost importance to the rest of my investigations.
- *Translocation* – and how this could be mastered through different sources and techniques, such as:
  - *plants*: some plants opened for spirits to enter the body and some plants hindered such access. Some plants even pushed pathological spirits into specific organs or parts of the body;
  - *vibrations and metals*: the use of vibrational bowls and metal plates to influence the spirits, usually to shift their place in the body to induce calm and pleasure, or to translocate them completely;

- ○ *metals taken internally*: ingestion of different metallic powders to translocate spirits – even the different parts of the spiritual make-up of the patients themselves so as to introduce a changed spirituality;
- ○ *acupuncture points*: the use of points on the body for the same reasons as described above, namely to manipulate pathological spirits, pathological parts of the patient's own spiritual make-up or parts of the spiritual sheaths of the patient, in order to introduce a changed perception of reality;
- ○ *movements*: different movements and postures could influence in the same way as described under 'acupuncture points' above.
- • *Transformation* – how a transformation relates to the three streams, and also to the morning–evening forces as opposed to the midday and midnight-forces;
- • *the direct stream of energy*: which furthers a transformation of the pathological entities;
- • *the morning–evening-forces:* which further the transformation of spiritual forces and entities in general.

Personal Comment

It is difficult for me to accept or to understand that this phenomenon of translocation – that is found within most kinds of contemporary medical systems and is so easy to observe – is not known or recognised by the various medical establishments in contemporary Western culture.

Whenever I lecture on this subject to colleagues, some Chinese doctor or veterinarian will stand up and tell the audience that this phenomenon is and has always been known very well in China.

The corruption of medicine and the subsequent triumph of Mammon is obvious to me and again very difficult to accept. I also have difficulty in understanding the blindness of my fellow doctors, healers, acupuncturists, homeopaths and veterinarians who don't see this. Finally, I have difficulties believing that many here in the West don't know this. Could it be that, due to money and power, they refrain from speaking the truth?

Chapter Four

*The demonic forces revealed during the midday–midnight
hours and their counterpart revealed during the morning–
evening hours in the secret temple of the emperor*

At the court, many people wondered, and there were
many secret discussions, about the identity of the spirit
speaking through the emperor. How did this spirit relate
to the legendary Yellow Emperor, who had lived or
incarnated hundreds of years before my own birth?

Most of the time our own emperor acted like a human
being, enjoying food and drink, women and the company of his royal friends. But at important moments
and times of decision, he completely changed. His face
became fiery, his speech became sharp, his countenance
became powerful and he expressed his opinions as if
from a superior intelligence.*

Also, when our emperor had delegated important
decisions or defensive military works to others, and they
were in the process of making these important decisions,
they too changed in a similar way. To us who lived and
worked at the royal court, it was obvious that at these
moments alien forces spoke through the emperor.

I myself once experienced this alien force when I was
determining the placement and function of our royal
sick-house (an early version of a hospital) – mainly for
the use of wounded soldiers and wealthy people. Our

---

* The same phenomenon has also been observed with other powerful
individuals, for example with Hitler when he gave significant speeches.

main camp, or city if we may call it so, was a short distance away from the Yellow River, close to the city that today is called Yuanyang, north of the Yellow River and north of today's Zhengzhou. I wanted us to build the main hospital on an island in the river directly south of our city, where our sick, wounded soldiers and doctors could be easily protected. I was appointed by the emperor's war chief to find a good place for the hospital, and had decided on this hidden island. As I was about to declare this decision, a strange power came over me; I had problems in talking, in seeing or in hearing and it was as if I was pushed out of my own body. I saw myself from above and heard myself saying that we must not place the hospital on an island in the river. We had to place the hospital on a nearby mountain, one day's journey directly north.

Then I clearly perceived the thinking behind this order. In a sense I was within the spirit that spoke, and could see through 'his' eyes and think through 'his' brain. I suddenly understood why we could not place the hospital on a river, due to the closeness to water. Water would hinder the translocation of the pathological demons, whilst if it were on a mountain – where the wind prevails – it would be easier. When I 'came back' into my own body, I was amazed and did not speak much for several days.

After this experience I decided to find out more about who this spirit was that ruled our lives, our thinking and our decisions in such a fundamental way. The only way to discover this was to find my way to the source of its power.

Behind the emperor's house was a secret and private temple, to which only the emperor and a few others had access. This temple was constructed in a very special way. It had a foundation on poles, lifted up from the ground, so that wind could circulate. The walls were bright red, and the roof ended in dragon-like figures. The roof was of the most special and interesting construction. It had five big holes in it with small roofs over each of them. The walls were made from about twelve layers of glass and gold. Inside the temple there were two rooms, one larger and one smaller, the latter having a huge statue of a dragon in it. Around the room there were seven slender pillars, holding up the roof. The floor consisted of three layers: a thick bottom layer, a thin middle layer and a normal walking floor as the upper and third layer. The emperor himself had given instructions as to its design.

I found out that it was possible to slip in between the second and third layers of the floor and there to hear all that was said. It was even possible to make a little hole at the end of this space so that I could see what was going on.

I hid in this secret temple that was meant only to be available to the emperor himself. After starting to understand the secrets of the three different energetic streams, and also having been able to lift the curse that had been put on my father, I had become so powerful that I considered it my right to do this. Also, maybe I could use what I learned to make myself even stronger – to know who and what the deeper force behind the Yang-demons was, and also what and who spoke through the emperor.

Almost every day around midday the emperor spent two hours in his secret and forbidden temple. In preparation I hid myself in the space beneath the floor. The experiences I then had in that temple almost made me go mad. I had been lying beneath the floor for several hours when the emperor arrived. It was about half an hour before midday. He had with him a servant who helped him with his clothes. All the clothes had to be changed into a costume made of silk with embroidered dragons. His usual head-adornment was removed. I seldom had seen him without this, as it symbolized his divine rank. He then drank a potion made up of different plants, anointed his head with an oil made from hemp, and started to sing.

Suddenly a spirit materialized above his head and descended into his body. The emperor's voice and whole appearance then changed as he began to speak. His personal servant wrote down what he said. I witnessed how the spirit of the old emperor spoke through the present emperor—or was it the voice of an even higher being?

The first time I witnessed this I was utterly shaken and frightened, but later I got used to this frightening scene as I often sneaked into the temple to listen to and to witness the commands given there. The voice gave instructions as to how to order society, how to heal diseases, how to produce weapons and medicines and much more.

I will now briefly describe some of the more important instructions given to the emperor through this materialized divinity which related to:

- The use of different frequencies through singing bowls and other instruments.
- The plants that could be used for different diseases, and also to be given to soldiers or women to make them obedient to the emperor's will.
- Procedures to make soldiers double their strength and life force.

- Acupuncture-points to regulate the hold of adversarial spirits, and how to translocate them.
- How to use different systems of pulse-diagnosis.
- Strategies for warfare.
- Times of the day when different duties should and should not be done. For example, it was forbidden to make any medicines, weapons or magic tools during three-hour periods in the mornings and evenings. These had to be produced in the middle of the day or in the middle of the night.

I spent a long time figuring out why it was forbidden to make important medicines, weapons or tools during the three hours in the morning and the evening (between 4 and 7 am and 4 and 7 pm). These secrets were not revealed to the emperor directly, and I only finally understood the reason through small clues.

At last I found out that the cosmic forces in the morning and the evening differed markedly from the cosmic forces governing midday and midnight. The morning forces were transformative, as the night was then transformed into something other, i.e. the rising sun of the day. The evening forces were also transformative, changing day into night.

Although this last change was conceived as not being good, it balanced the transformation that occurred in the morning. These two forces supported a transformation that was considered to be highly undesirable, as one of the most important laws in China then – as now – was to secure the stability of the system, the status quo.

The cosmic forces dominant at midday and at midnight did not help transformation, rather the opposite. They supported stability, not change, and this furthered translocation, which implied no change except for the habitat of the demons. The most effective time to trans-locate a disease – a demon of the luciferic type – was in the middle of the day or in the middle of the night. Treating patients during the morning or evening was forbidden. The experiences of treating with acupuncture in the morning, compared to midday, was described and elaborated at length. This seemed to be very important.

Another secret that I tried to understand was the true identity of the legendary Yellow Emperor, the present emperor as well as the force that spoke through both. This was the most interesting information I gleaned from my secret period of time in the hidden chamber beneath the floor. The Yellow Emperor was not a human being but an empty shell of an individual that had not incarnated before. In this shell a mighty spirit came in and out. This mighty spirit was named 'the Yellow God', 'the Deity from Below', 'the Dragon master', 'the Dragon' or other similar titles. This 'deity' was mighty, shining and full of wisdom.

Based on the strong avoidance of any transforming force, I started to understand the quality of this force or 'deity'. It wanted no change, but instead desired that humanity went on forever, following the same rules and the same system. In other words, this 'deity' simply wanted a circular history, so that everything repeated itself over and over again—to return to old habits, old rules and to keep everything as it was.

Today we know this being under the name of Lucifer – a being that has been with humankind for a very long time. In every cycle of time, this 'deity' has changed, especially its colours. Although it hates any form of change, of course it has had to follow the general evolution of both time and space, as well as of humanity itself. It therefore always tries to hinder true evolution, as it hates all kinds of transformation. Even so, it changes its colours for every cycle of time.

Also, I observed that the colours that the 'deity' adopted when speaking about various periods of time, reflected the very colours that stemmed from those periods. For example, when the 'deity' gave information relating to the ancient world of Hyperborea, this transfer of knowledge glowed in a yellow light. In the Lemurian period, the whole room glowed as from a pink light. Atlantean information – which preceded the Chinese culture and from which most knowledge of that period came – glowed brownish-red. When speaking about the period 4,000 years ago, the information given glowed a bright red.

Chapter Five

Warfare and magical war-techniques. Death of the emperor.
Leaving of the controlling spirit

Since time immemorial, internal war had been waged in the Middle Kingdom, which today we call China. Different clans, families, groups or small kingdoms have always striven for dominion.

Before 3101 BC, these wars were fought in close relationship to the spiritual worlds and laws, based mainly on the good forces, the higher hierarchies and spirits.

After 3101, and especially after the incarnation of Lucifer as the Yellow Emperor, increasingly warfare was fought in relation to and with the support of luciferic adversarial forces, and the war-techniques became crueller and more devastating.[*]

As a doctor at the royal court, I was not so much involved in the war itself, but I had the responsibility for nursing and treating the wounded – and also, as we will see, the preparation of the 'special soldiers' who spread so much fear and suffering at that time.[†]

Signs of a coming war – one more in an endless stream of violence – were at hand. Three of the neighbouring provinces or clans had been growing in wealth and power, and had been preparing for war with an extensive

---

[*] Today war-techniques are becoming more and more influenced by the ahrimanic forces, i.e. they are exceedingly technical.

[†] Today this work has also been shifted from the luciferic to the ahrimanic, as even robot soldiers are now being developed, with a great capacity to kill and destroy.

production of weapons. My emperor also made extensive preparations for war, and I was ordered to organize the medical rescue team and prepare new and fresh soldiers.

The 'special soldiers' came to be feared throughout the area, and later gave rise to myths that some of them were immortal. This was partly true and partly not true, as they *could* be killed, although with great difficulty.

The preparation of such soldiers was partly done with my help, as well as the help of other doctors and healers skilled in translocation techniques. The final preparation reminded me of 'ordinary' healing. This preparation was completely different to the usual treatment of ordinary disease by means of translocation, although the techniques were fundamentally the same.

This was a quite new technique in that period, although it had also been used before the destruction of the Atlantean civilization, and several of us had a distant memory of this. In Atlantis there was much experimenting with projecting thought-forms into physical matter, animals, humans or even 'half-human' forms. These thought-forms could especially strengthen those who received a 'warrior thought-form'.

For some time I had been experimenting with the translocation of life-forces in the form of thought-forms, both between other people and between them and myself. In this way I had been able to create soldiers with double etheric strength that were capable of extreme endurance and as a consequence were almost impossible to kill.

In our present culture a faint echo of this can be seen when soldiers take large quantities of drugs like cocaine or amphetamines. If they are hurt or wounded, they seem to have greater stamina than one would expect. This has to do with the adversarial spirit that is channelled into the soldier's body via the spiritual portals that are opened up with the use of drugs.

Another method was to translocate the etheric body of a prisoner to one of our own soldiers, in order to make him twice as strong. This last method was the best, easiest and most durable. The prisoner would then of course die a painful death, having only an astral body left – a body that would feel all kinds of pain due to his missing – stolen – etheric body. But we did not care about that! With the mentality we had, the sufferings of one individual were of no importance to us.

In the film *Lord of the Rings*, knowledge of such soldiers is reflected in the so-called 'Uruk-hai'. Even the name of these indefatigable soldiers of Saruman is very much like the name we used in ancient China for the soldiers with such a 'double etheric body'. We called them *Xia Ruak-Hi*. They received this name because they were 'invented' during the Xia-dynasty – or actually some years before the founding of this dynasty, in the pre-dynastic time.

These soldiers were used in this war, and we won it with ease as our enemies were stunned and fearful when encountering such men that were almost impossible to kill. Even if they were pierced with an arrow or a spear, these 'special' soldiers just went on fighting. The word soon spread that as an army we were invincible, and then almost all resistance stopped.

The work with these soldiers, and the victories we had in our wars, made my own power, as well as my use of black magic, greater than ever. I even had a bodyguard of these fearsome worriers of the *Xia Ruak-Hi*. This made me dangerous in the eyes of all, including the emperor.

Chapter Six

Degradation and murder

Within the inner circles of the court, a growing discontent with my ever-stronger position had developed. Even the emperor himself did not like it when anyone became too powerful – although they could never become as strong as he was, as an instrument for Lucifer.

Having from time to time felt 'the Ancient One' – the old Yellow Emperor – within me and speaking through me, and having felt the power of his light with its concomitant knowledge and abilities, made me feel hubris – a hubris that in the end was to cause my death.

I was supported by my personal and magical body-guard *Xia Ruak-Hi*, and this also gave me a false sense of safety and security.

The skills I had developed during the last war had made me dangerous, as I could now translocate my own thought-forms to others, and I could also translocate the etheric forces between two human beings, so that one of them got strong whilst the other died.

*

In my present incarnation I have seen remnants of this phenomenon many times, for example with experiments done within both homeopathy and acupuncture where two animals with the same disease are treated, one with conventional medicine and the other with alternative methods. The one treated conventionally might die after three days whilst the other is cured. The explanation for this is simple enough, although usually the person conducting the experiment has no knowledge of the inner dynamics of what is happening.

When an animal is treated with herbs, homeopathy or acupuncture, the translocation of the pathological demon or demonic power takes about three days. As the other animal already has a weak area which contains a pathological demon, the translocated demon from the other creature can easily slip in. The animal treated with conventional medicine ends up having two somewhat similar demons. (The translocation of demons in patients who are treated with conventional medicine takes around three weeks.)

The poor animal with two demons then has to try to survive for three more weeks, and that is often too much. That is why it dies more easily when in proximity with another animal treated for the same disease using alternative medicine.

It is quite strange how these old procedures and techniques can suddenly show up thousands of years later – actually, tens of thousands of years later! They were first developed in old Atlantis, then rejuvenated in ancient China and finally a memory of it shows up in today's medical experiments relating to the efficacy of acupuncture, herbs or homeopathy in relation to conventional medicine.

*

Returning to my story, I clearly understood that I was now in a dangerous position. What I did not know was that both the emperor and the group of secondary doctors serving at the court were plotting against me.

One day, on my way back to the emperor's castle and court, I was ambushed and captured by several strong men. As I had left my bodyguard behind, I was unable to defend myself. The perpetrators took me to a small cottage in the nearby forest where I was left.

I counted on my bodyguards to rescue me, and also on my strong magical powers to fight my enemies, but I was wrong. My enemies had engaged a very powerful sorcerer, and through secret rituals my powers were taken away from me by the technique of 'reversed initiation'.

This ritual technique was performed in a way I myself had used in my time as an oracle in Atlantis.* It was performed with the 'tie' method, when a magical string was tied around the throat, hindering all three streams of etheric power from entering the body, especially the hands. These forces entered through the sense-organs of the head and from here continued through the body as earlier described. These forces or powers were and still are essential for performing all kinds of healing, magic or dark magic.

In this way I lost the ability to heal, the power to translocate as well as other magic skills. This power was related to the hands, as they channelled the force taken in through the head. The kundalini-power rising upwards was also used in this work, but all forces were hindered by the magic string. This procedure was performed with the help of both my friends and my wife. Oh, how I hated those who made me endure this!

These rituals of reversed initiation took three days to perform and I was then released from the cabin. Now I was without my magical powers or my bodyguards, as

---

* Described in my book *The Forgotten Mysteries of Atlantis.*

their loyalty and strength depended on me still having my strength and my magic abilities.

A few days later I took my revenge – not through magic or the use of my bodyguards, but through cold-blooded murder. I attacked the three leading plotters with a sword and knife and I killed them all, including my wife. Later, the murders were discovered and I received my deserved punishment.

Chapter Seven

Death and reincarnation

After I had murdered the three most prominent members of the group of doctors attached to the imperial court as well as my own wife, the emperor's judges took me to court in order to sentence me to death.

The court 'witnessed' that I had been taken hold of by luciferic forces – by Lucifer himself. The spirit of the old emperor did not only speak through me, as most of the members of the court had witnessed themselves; no, the spirit took total hold of me, changing me from who I was to the old emperor! This was a sin whose wages were death. Only the emperor was allowed fully to channel the old emperor – the Yellow Emperor, Lucifer himself.

A board was summoned in secret, and this matter was discussed. The 'Great Spirit' had taken total hold of someone other than the emperor himself, which had never been seen before during the 600-year period since the death of the original Yellow Emperor. Therefore, they discussed how to eliminate me, as they considered me quite dangerous. This was difficult as the emperor was quite sick at that time, and I was needed in order to keep him alive. However, it soon became evident that I had lost my healing powers and therefore I could easily be sentenced to death, as the emperor no longer had need of me. Also, I was no longer dangerous, having lost both my powers and my bodyguards, so in the eyes of my enemies it was better to eliminate me totally.

In their view, I should be hindered from reincarnating, as they feared that I still had my knowledge and as such could be dangerous in a later incarnation.

A death sentence was passed, in the same way as the death sentence had been passed on my father, 33 years before. I was sentenced to drink a poison, thus killing myself with the extract of bitter almonds.

I knew that doing this would be extremely detrimental to my future being. All my black deeds would be cast back on me and, with my etheric mirror shattered, it would be impossible to work with my karma and regain the possibility for future incarnations.

I had to find a solution to this problem. Finally, a scheme to avoid this dark and discouraging future presented itself to me. I was taken to the house where all prisoners of higher backgrounds were incarcerated before an execution, and on the way to this house we passed a horse guard. I jumped out behind the horse, kicking it as hard as I could. The expected reaction came immediately. I was dead a fraction of a second later, killed by the horse's violent kick. Thus I died, killed by a horse, ready to work with my difficult karma in many incarnations to follow.

Conclusion

Our present world has deep roots arising from ancient deeds of black magic. These roots are partly collective, partly individual.

In old Atlantis I was personally responsible for some very dark deeds – deeds that echoed down through several of my later incarnations, finding an especially fertile ground in my Chinese incarnation 4,000 years ago at the court of the emperor.

As we have seen, during this period, from 2500 BC until around the time of the birth of Christ, the emperors of China were heavily influenced by the Yellow Emperor, who was actually the vessel for Lucifer himself. These emperors laid the foundation for the medical, political and religious–philosophical systems that promote luciferic powers, systems and entities, including demons and elementals.

The change to a five-element system, as well as the merging of Yin and Yang, make possible the enduring existence of pathological entities called luciferic- or Yang-elemental structures. These changes enabled these entities to cause pathology and disease through the process of translocation – to wherever or to whoever they wanted to go.

This book draws these historical and personal threads all the way from Atlantis through the ancient Chinese culture and ending in our modern-day medical systems.

May this book be a contribution to enabling humanity to find the way from translocation to transformation.

Appendix

A timeline to the deception and to healing impulses

8000–3101 years BC
Most diseases were healed with transformation, but from quite other powers than the Christ force.

3101 years BC
The general clairvoyance was lost as the cosmos entered *Kali Yuga*. This made the hiding of translocation possible.

2666 years BC
The incarnation of Lucifer in China as the Yellow Emperor.

2666–2000 years BC
Extensive work and development of the five-elements and of pulse positions.

2000 years BC
My incarnation at the royal court, and extensive work and development relating to the five-elements and pulse positions.

AD 29–33
The eternal healing impulse, the Christ, is incarnated in the middle of the earth, in Palestine. Jesus healed people in twenty-four different ways, relating to the twelve zodiacal signs connected to the two adversarial forces.

AD 1899
The dark age, *Kali Yuga*, ends and the new Age of Light begins. A major change in the earth's etheric layer takes place, and all medicine, medical herbs and healing has to be revised.

AD 1900–1944
Peter Deunov, the world Master, presented his view of diseases, and fully acknowledged the phenomenon of translocation.

AD 1900–1923
Rudolf Steiner introduced the consciousness of the Middle-Point, the Christ-consciousness, the importance of the twelvefold zodiac and the threefold nature of the universe and the human being.

AD 1933
The etheric Christ-force appears in the etheric world, thus making it possible to heal by means of transformation out of the etheric body.

AD 2019 years
A new understanding of transformation and translocation appears.

AD 2000–2333 years
The incarnation of the being of Ahriman in America.

Books to challenge **ⓒ** *your perception of reality*

A message from Clairview

We are an independent publishing company with a focus on cutting-edge, non-fiction books. Our innovative list covers current affairs and politics, health, the arts, history, science and spirituality. But regardless of subject, our books have a common link: they all question conventional thinking, dogmas and received wisdom.

Despite being a small company, our list features some big names, such as Booker Prize winner Ben Okri, literary giant Gore Vidal, world leader Mikhail Gorbachev, modern artist Joseph Beuys and natural childbirth pioneer Michel Odent.

So, check out our full catalogue online at
www.clairviewbooks.com
and join our emailing list for news on new titles.

office@clairviewbooks.com

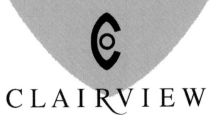

CLAIRVIEW